Juicing Recipe Book

for Beginners

The 50 Top Recipes to Stay Fit and

Lose Weight

Ally Stewart

information presented, whether for breach of contract, tort, negligence, personal injury, criminal intent, or under any other cause of action.

You agree to accept all risks of using the information presented inside this book.

You agree that by continuing to read this book, where appropriate and/or necessary, you shall consult a professional (including but not limited to your doctor, attorney, or financial advisor or such other advisor as needed) before using any of the suggested remedies, techniques, or information in this book.

Table of Contents

Introduction

When you're looking for a healthy way to feel energized for the day, you should consider making a smoothie at home. You'll be amazed at how quickly you can get the nutritional benefits of fresh fruit and vegetables without all the fuss of preparing it yourself. There's no reason why you should suffer again when making smoothies is so easy!

While Smoothies are extremely easy and quick to prepare, sometimes, even if you have the best intention, luck does not stay with you and as a result, Smoothies do end up being unsavory. Or perhaps just simply due to lack of time, you aren't able to make one.

There are certain tips and tricks for situations such as these that will allow you to batch prep the ingredients for your Smoothies beforehand so that you are able to make your Smoothie in seconds after you wake up in the morning.

A good prep pathway includes:

- Make sure to properly wash, prep and measure out your ingredients before making smoothies.

- Make sure to add ingredients in a baggie jar, seal and label them with smoothie name.

- Once you are ready to sip, pour the liquid into a blender and dump all the contents of your bag into the blender and blend well.

The number of smoothie kits that you create will largely depend on the free space that you have in your freezer. But you can create at least 5 smoothie kits for your 4 days of the week, which should be a good place to start.

Another option is to fully blend your smoothie, make it and then just freeze it into cubes.

Smoothies 1

Kale Smoothie

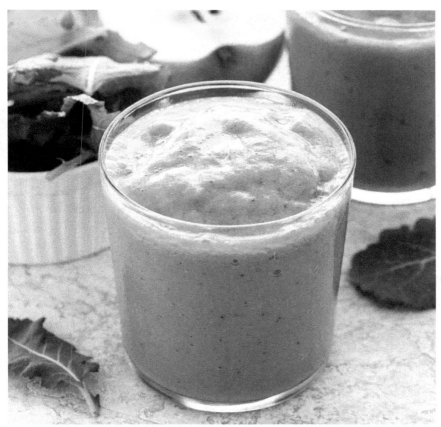

Preparation Time: 5 minutes

Cooking Time: 0 minutes

Servings: 2

Ingredients:

- 2 cups chopped kale leaves
- 1 banana, peeled
- 1 cup frozen strawberries
- 1 cup unsweetened almond milk
- 4 Medjool dates, pitted and chopped

Directions:

1. Put all the ingredients in a food processor, then blitz until glossy and smooth.
2. Serve immediately or chill in the refrigerator for an hour before serving.

Nutrition:

Calories: 663

Fat: 10.0g

Carbs: 142.5g

Fiber: 19.0g

Protein: 17.4g

Hot Tropical Smoothie

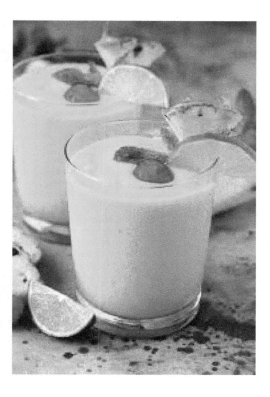

Preparation Time: 5 minutes

Cooking Time: 0 minutes

Servings: 4

 Ingredients:

- 1 cup frozen mango chunks
- 1 cup frozen pineapple chunks

- 1 small tangeri ne, peeled and pitted
- 2 cups spinach leaves
- 1 cup coconut water
- ¼ teaspoon cayenne pepper, optional

Directions:

1. Add all the ingredients in a food processor, then blitz until the mixture is smooth and combine well.
2. Serve immediately or chill in the refrigerator for an hour before serving.

Nutrition:

Calories: 283

Fat: 1.9g

Carbs: 67.9g

Fiber: 10.4g

Protein: 6.4g

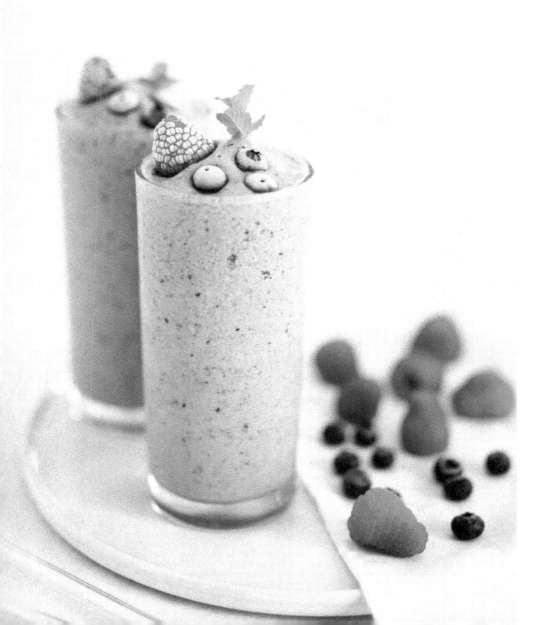

Berry Smoothie

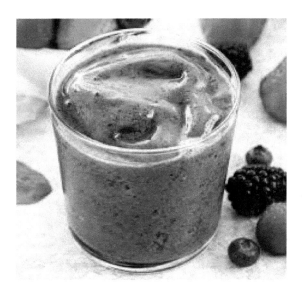

Preparation Time: 5 minutes

Cooking Time: 0 minutes

Servings: 4

 Ingredients:

- 1 cup berry mix (strawberries, blueberries, and cranberries)
- 4 Medjool dates, pitted and chopped
- 1½ cups unsweetened almond milk, plus more as needed

 Directions:

Add all the ingredients in a blender, then process until the mixture is smooth and well mixed.

Serve immediately or chill in the refrigerator for an hour before serving.

Nutrition:

Calories: 473

Fat: 4.0g

Carbs: 103.7g

Fiber: 9.7g

Protein: 14.8g

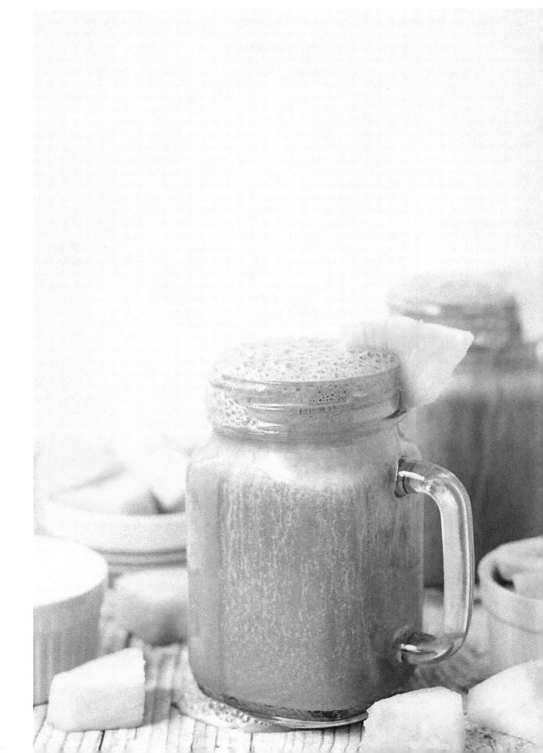

Cranberry and Banana Smoothie

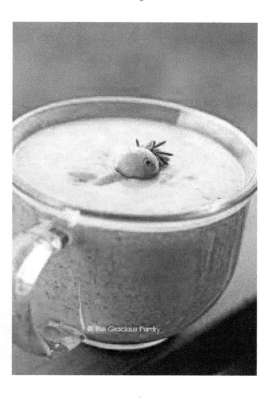

Preparation Time: 5 minutes

Cooking Time: 0 minutes

Servings: 4

Ingredients:

- 1 cup frozen cranberries
- 1 large banana, peeled

- 4 Medjool dates, pitted and chopped
- 1½ cups unsweetened almond milk

Directions:

Add all the ingredients in a food processor, then process until the mixture is glossy and well mixed.

Serve immediately or chill in the refrigerator for an hour before serving.

Nutrition:

Calories: 616

Fat: 8.0g

Carbs: 132.8g

Fiber: 14.6g

Protein: 15.7g

Pumpkin Smoothie

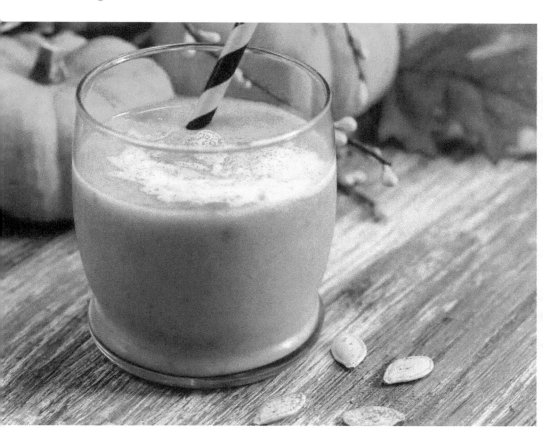

Preparation Time: 5 minutes

Cooking Time: 0 minutes

Servings: 5

Ingredients:

- ½ cup pumpkin purée
- 4 Medjool dates, pitted and chopped
- 1 cup unsweetened almond milk
- ¼ teaspoon vanilla extract
- ¼ teaspoon ground cinnamon
- ½ cup ice
- Pinch ground nutmeg

Directions:

Add all the ingredients in a blender, then process until the mixture is glossy and well mixed.

Serve immediately.

Nutrition:

Calories: 417

Fat: 3.0g

Carbs: 94.9g

Fiber: 10.4g

Protein: 11.4g

Super Smoothie

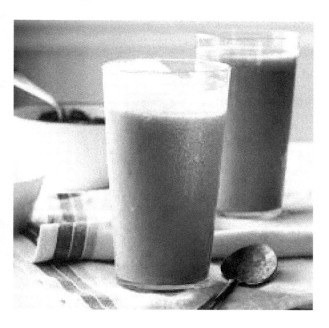

Preparation Time: 5 minutes

Cooking Time: 0 minutes

Servings: 4

Ingredients:

- 1 banana, peeled
- 1 cup chopped mango
- 1 cup raspberries
- ¼ cup rolled oats
- 1 carrot, peeled

- 1 cup chopped fresh kale
- 2 tablespoons chopped fresh parsley
- 1 tablespoon flaxseeds
- 1 tablespoon grated fresh ginger
- ½ cup unsweetened soy milk
- 1 cup water

Directions:

Put all the ingredients in a food processor, then blitz until glossy and smooth.

Serve immediately or chill in the refrigerator for an hour before serving.

Nutrition:

Calories: 550

Fat: 39.0g

Carbs: 31.0g

Fiber: 15.0g

Protein: 13.0g

Kiwi and Strawberry Smoothie

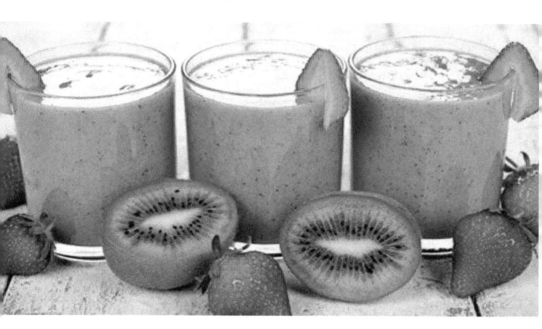

Preparation Time: 5 minutes

Cooking Time: 0 minutes

Servings: 3

Ingredients:

- 1 kiwi, peeled
- 5 medium strawberries
- ½ frozen banana
- 1 cup unsweetened almond milk

- 2 tablespoons hemp seeds
- 2 tablespoons peanut butter
- 1 to 2 teaspoons maple syrup
- ½ cup spinach leaves
- Handful broccoli sprouts

Directions:

Put all the ingredients in a food processor, then blitz until creamy and smooth.

Serve immediately or chill in the refrigerator for an hour before serving.

Nutrition:

Calories: 562

Fat: 28.6g

Carbs: 63.6g

Fiber: 15.1g

Protein: 23.3g

Banana and Chai Chia Smoothie

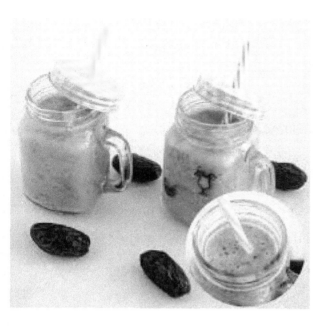

Preparation Time: 5 minutes

Cooking Time: 0 minutes

Servings: 3

Ingredients:

- 1 banana
- 1 cup alfalfa sprouts
- 1 tablespoon chia seeds

- ½ cup unsweetened coconut milk
- 1 to 2 soft Medjool dates, pitted
- ¼ teaspoon ground cinnamon
- 1 tablespoon grated fresh ginger
- 1 cup water
- Pinch ground cardamom

Directions:

Add all the ingredients in a blender, then process until the mixture is smooth and creamy. Add water or coconut milk if necessary.

Serve immediately.

Nutrition:

Calories: 477

Fat: 41.0g

Carbs: 31.0g

Fiber: 14.0g

Protein: 8.0g

Chocolate and Peanut Butter Smoothie

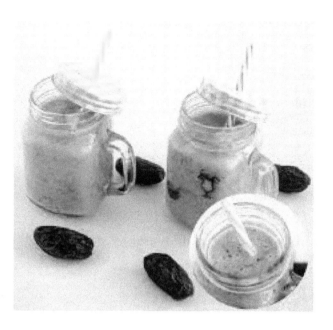

Preparation Time: 5 minutes

Cooking Time: 0 minutes

Servings: 4

Ingredients:

- 1 tablespoon unsweetened cocoa powder
- 1 tablespoon peanut butter
- 1 banana

- 1 teaspoon maca powder
- ½ cup unsweetened soy milk
- ¼ cup rolled oats
- 1 tablespoon flaxseeds
- 1 tablespoon maple syrup
- 1 cup water

Directions:

Add all the ingredients in a blender, then process until the mixture is smooth and creamy. Add water or soy milk if necessary.

Serve immediately.

Nutrition:

Calories: 474

Fat: 16.0g

Carbs: 27.0g

Fiber: 18.0g

Protein: 13.0g

Golden Milk

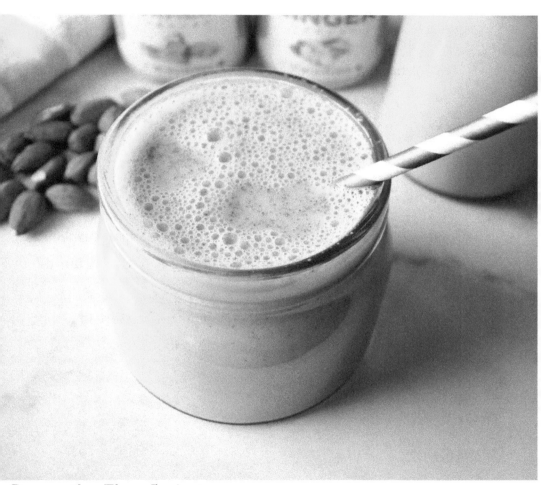

Preparation Time: 5 minutes

Cooking Time: 0 minutes

Servings: 4

Ingredients:

- ¼ teaspoon ground cinnamon
- ½ teaspoon ground turmeric
- ½ teaspoon grated fresh ginger
- 1 teaspoon maple syrup
- 1 cup unsweetened coconut milk
- Ground black pepper, to taste
- 2 tablespoon water

Directions:

Combine all the ingredients in a saucepan. Stir to mix well.
Heat over medium heat for 5 minutes. Keep stirring during
the heating.
Allow to cool for 5 minutes, then pour the mixture in a
blender. Pulse until creamy and smooth. Serve
immediately.

Nutrition:

Calories: 577

Fat: 57.3g

Carbs: 19.7g

Fiber: 6.1g

Protein: 5.7g

Mango Agua Fresca

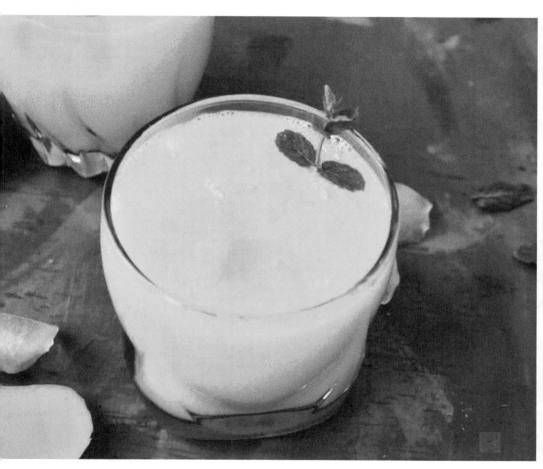

Preparation Time: 5 minutes

Cooking Time: 0 minutes

Servings: 2

Ingredients:

- 2 fresh mangoes, diced
- 1½ cups water
- 1 teaspoon fresh lime juice
- Maple syrup, to taste
- 2 cups ice
- 2 slices fresh lime, for garnish
- 2 fresh mint sprigs, for garnish

Directions:

Put the mangoes, lime juice, maple syrup, and water in a blender. Process until creamy and smooth.

Divide the beverage into two glasses, then garnish each glass with ice, lime slice, and mint sprig before serving.

Nutrition:

Calories: 230

Fat: 1.3g

Carbs: 57.7g

Fiber: 5.4g

Protein: 2.8g

Light Ginger Tea

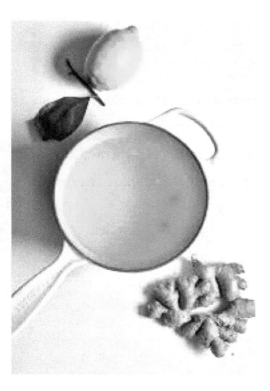

Preparation Time: 5 minutes

Cooking Time: 10 to 15 minutes

Servings: 2

Ingredients:

- 1 small ginger knob, sliced into four 1-inch chunks
- 4 cups water

- Juice of 1 large lemon
- Maple syrup, to taste

Directions:

Add the ginger knob and water in a saucepan, then simmer over medium heat for 10 to 15 minutes.

Turn off the heat, then mix in the lemon juice. Strain the liquid to remove the ginger, then fold in the maple syrup and serve.

Nutrition:

Calories: 32

Fat: 0.1g

Carbs: 8.6g

Fiber: 0.1g

Protein: 0.1g

Classic Switchel

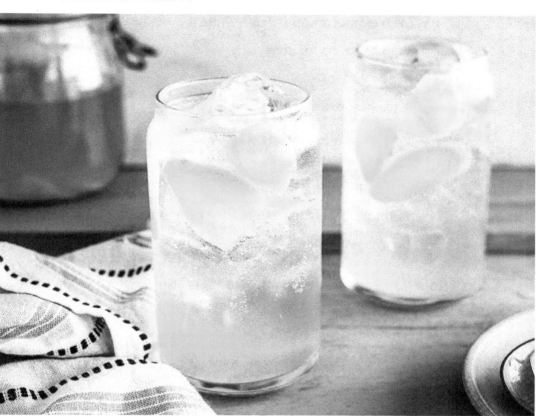

Preparation Time: 5 minutes

Cooking Time: 0 minutes

Servings: 4

Ingredients:

- 1-inch piece ginger, minced
- 2 tablespoons apple cider vinegar
- 2 tablespoons maple syrup
- 4 cups water
- ¼ teaspoon sea salt, optional

Directions:

Combine all the ingredients in a glass. Stir to mix well. Serve immediately or chill in the refrigerator for an hour before serving.

Nutrition:

Calories: 110

Fat: 0g

Carbs: 28.0g

Fiber: 0g

Protein: 0g

Lime and Cucumber Electrolyte Drink

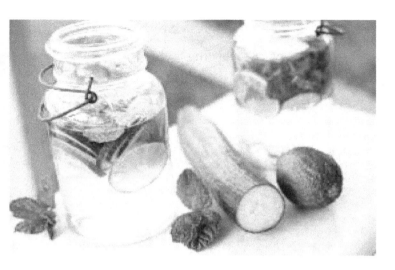

Preparation Time: 5 minutes

Cooking Time: 0 minutes

Servings: 4

Ingredients:

- ¼ cup chopped cucumber
- 1 tablespoon fresh lime juice
- 1 tablespoon apple cider vinegar
- 2 tablespoons maple syrup
- ¼ teaspoon sea salt, optional
- 4 cups water

Directions:

Combine all the ingredients in a glass. Stir to mix well. Refrigerate overnight before serving.

Nutrition:

Calories: 114

Fat: 0.1g

Carbs: 28.9g

Fiber: 0.3g

Protein: 0.3g

Easy and Fresh Mango Madness

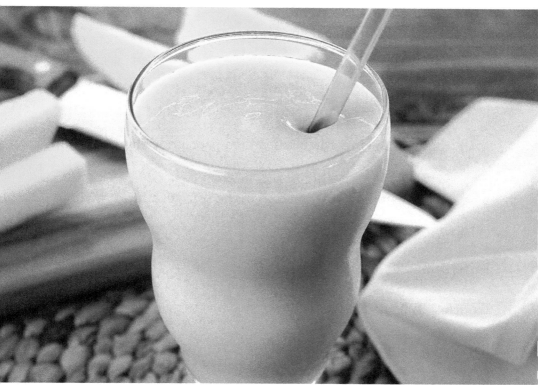

Preparation Time: 5 minutes

Cooking Time: 0 minutes

Servings: 4

Ingredients:

- 1 cup chopped mango
- 1 cup chopped peach

- 1 banana
- 1 cup strawberries
- 1 carrot, peeled and chopped
- 1 cup water

Directions:

Put all the ingredients in a food processor, then blitz until glossy and smooth.

Serve immediately or chill in the refrigerator for an hour before serving.

Nutrition:

Calories: 376

Fat: 22.0g

Carbs: 19.0g

Fiber: 14.0g

Protein: 5.0g

Simple Date Shake

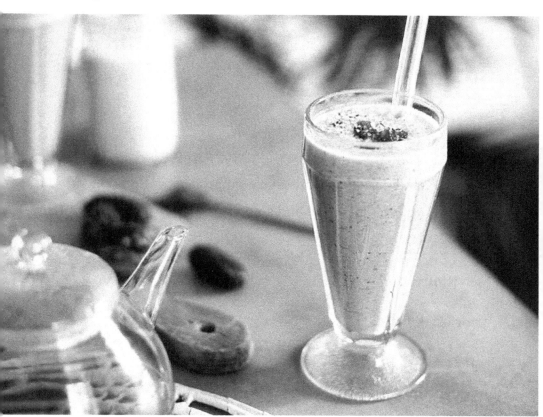

Preparation Time: 10 minutes

Cooking Time: 0 minutes

Servings: 2

Ingredients:

- 5 Medjool dates, pitted, soaked in boiling water for 5 minutes

- ¾ cup unsweetened coconut milk
- 1 teaspoon vanilla extract
- ½ teaspoon fresh lemon juice
- ¼ teaspoon sea salt, optional
- 1½ cups ice

Directions:

Put all the ingredients in a food processor, then blitz until it has a milkshake and smooth texture.

Serve immediately.

Nutrition:

Calories: 380

Fat: 21.6g

Carbs: 50.3g

Fiber: 6.0g

Protein: 3.2g

Beet and Clementine Protein Smoothie

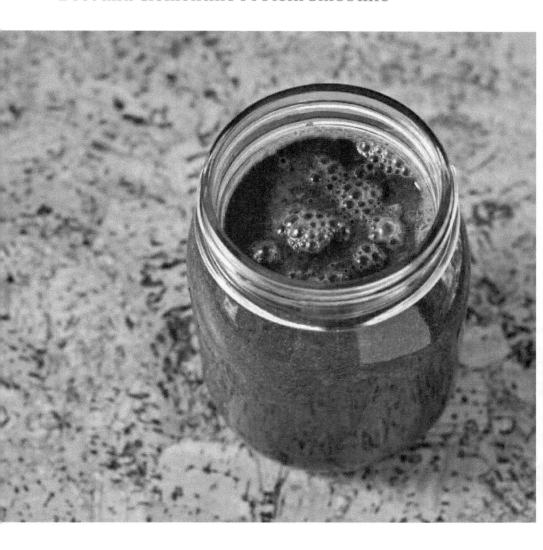

Preparation Time: 10 minutes

Cooking Time: 0 minutes

Servings: 3

Ingredients:

- 1 small beet, peeled and chopped
- 1 clementine, peeled and broken into segments
- ½ ripe banana
- ½ cup raspberries
- 1 tablespoon chia seeds
- 2 tablespoons almond butter
- ¼ teaspoon vanilla extract
- 1 cup unsweetened almond milk
- 1/8 teaspoon fine sea salt, optional

Directions:

Combine all the ingredients in a food processor, then pulse on high for 2 minutes or until glossy and creamy.

Refrigerate for an hour and serve chilled.

Nutrition:

Calories: 526; Fat: 25.4g; Carbs: 61.9g; Fiber: 17.3g; Protein: 20.6g

Matcha Limeade

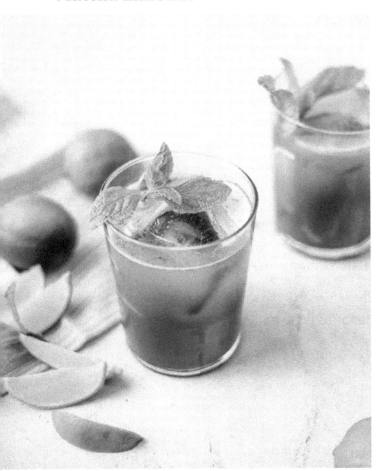

Preparation Time: 10 minutes

Cooking Time: 0 minutes

Servings: 4

Ingredients:

2 tablespoons matcha powder

¼ cup raw agave syrup

3 cups water, divided

1 cup fresh lime juice

3 tablespoons chia seeds

Directions:

Lightly simmer the matcha, agave syrup, and 1 cup of water in a saucepan over medium heat. Keep stirring until no matcha lumps.

Pour the matcha mixture in a large glass, then add the remaining ingredients and stir to mix well.

Refrigerate for at least an hour before serving.

Nutrition:

Calories: 152

Fat: 4.5g

Carbs: 26.8g

Fiber: 5.3g

Protein: 3.7g

Green & Mean

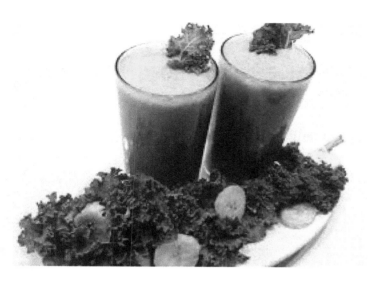

Preparation time: 10 minutes

Cooking time: 0 minutes

Servings: 1

Ingredients:

- 3 stalks of Celery
- 3 bunches of Kale
- 1/2 cup of sliced pineapple
- 1/2 apple, chopped
- A handful of spinach
- 1 tablespoon of coconut oil

- 1 scoop of vanilla Protein powder

Directions:

Place all the **Ingredients** together in the blender and process until the desired consistency is achieved.

Pour contents of the blender into a tall glass.

Serve immediately and enjoy!

Nutrition:

Calories: 497

Protein: 28g

Carbs: 62g

Fat: 17g

Chocolate Peanut Delight

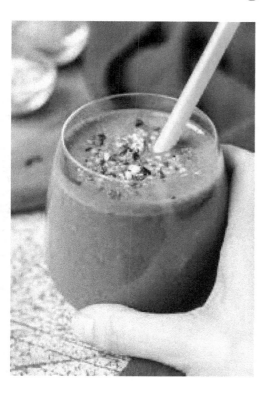

Preparation time: 10 minutes

Cooking time: 0 minutes

Servings: 1

Ingredients:

- 1 scoop of chocolate whey Protein powder
- 1 cup of low-Fat Greek yog urt

- 1 whole banana
- 2 tablespoon of peanut butter
- 1 cup of ice

Directions:

Add all the ingredients to a blender and blend until smooth

Enjoy

Nutrition:

Calories: 656

Protein: 63g

Carbs: 55g

Fat: 21g

Smoothies 2

Amy's Homemade Mass Gainer

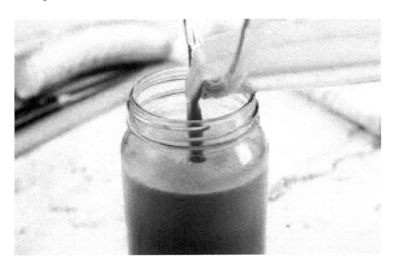

Preparation time: 10 minutes

Cooking time: 0 minutes

Servings: 1

Ingredients:

- 2 scoop of chocolate whey Protein powder
- 2 cups of whole milk
- 1/2 cup of dry rolled oats
- 1 whole banana
- 2 tablespoon of organic almond butter

- 1 cup of crushed ice

Directions:

Add all the ingredients to a blender and blend until smooth

Enjoy

Nutrition

Calories: 970

Protein: 75g

Carbs: 90g

Fat: 30g

Berry Protein Shake

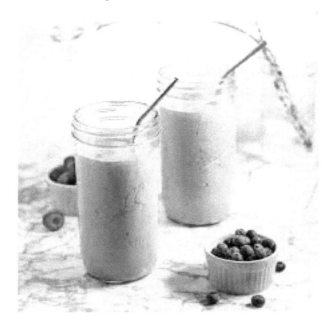

Preparation time: 10 minutes

Cooking time: 0 minutes

Servings: 1

Ingredients:

- 2 scoop of whey Protein powder
- 1 cup of blueberries
- 1 cup of blackberries
- 1 cup of raspberries
- 1 cup of water   1 cup of ice

Directions:

Add all the ingredients to a blender and blend until smooth

Enjoy

Nutrition:

Calories: 342

Protein: 38g

Carbs: 42g

Fat: 3g

Fresh Strawberry Shake

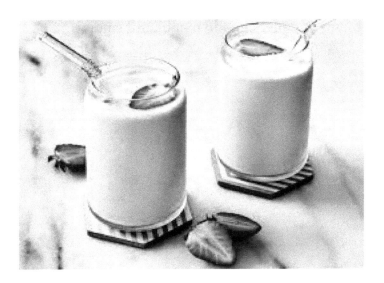

Preparation time: 10 minutes

Cooking time: 0 minutes

Servings: 1

Ingredients:

- 2 scoops of vanilla Protein powder
- 1 cup of strawberries
- 2 cups of water
- 1 tablespoon of flaxseed oil

Directions:

Add all the ingredients to a blender and blend until smooth

Enjoy

Nutrition:

Calories: 303

Protein: 35g

Carbs: 15g

Fat: 11g

Choco Coffee Energy Shake

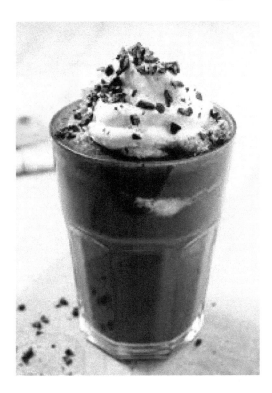

Preparation time: 10 minutes

Cooking time: 0 minutes

Servings: 1

Ingredients:

- 2 scoops of chocolate Protein powder
- 1/2 cup of l ow-Fat milk

- 1 cup of water
- 1 tablespoon of instant coffee

Directions:

Add all the ingredients to a blender and blend until smooth

Enjoy

Nutrition:

Calories: 299

Protein: 42g

Carbs: 14g

Fat: 6g

Lean and Mean Pineapple Shake

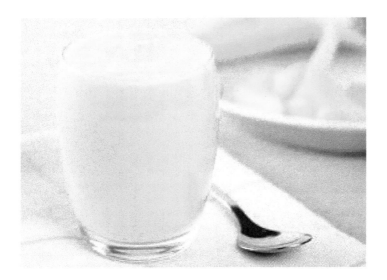

Preparation time: 10 minutes

Cooking time: 0 minutes

Servings: 1

Ingredients:

- 1 cup chopped fresh pineapple
- 4 strawberries
- 1 banana
- 1 tablespoon low-Fat Greek yogurt
- 1 scoop of vanilla Protein powder
- 1 cup of water

Directions:

Add all the ingredients to a blender and blend until smooth.

Enjoy

Nutrition

Calories: 355

Protein: 23g

Carbs: 65g

Fat: 3g

Chopped Almond Smoothie

Preparation time: 10 minutes

Cooking time: 0 minutes

Servings: 1

Ingredients:

- 1 1/2 cups water
- 17 chopped almonds
- 1/2 teaspoon coconut extract
- 1 scoop chocolate Protein powder

Directions:

Add all the ingredients to a blender and blend until smooth

Enjoy

Nutrition:

Calories: 241

Protein: 24g

Carbs: 6g

Fat: 13g

Vanilla Strawberry Surprise

Preparation time: 10 minutes

Cooking time: 0 minutes

Servings: 1

Ingredients:

- 2 scoops of vanilla Protein powder
- 1 cup of ice
- 1 banana
- 4 fresh or frozen strawberries

Directions:

Add all the ingredients to a blender and blend until smooth.

Enjoy

Nutrition:

Calories: 329

Protein: 36g

Carbs: 42g

Fat: 2g

Breakfast Banana Shake

Preparation time: 10 minutes

Cooking time: 0 minutes

Servings: 1

Ingredients:

- 3/4 cup of low-Fat milk
- 1 banana
- 1/4 pound of rolled oats
- 2 scoops of vanilla whey Protein powder

Directions:

Add all the ingredients to a blender and blend until smooth

Enjoy

Nutrition:

Calories: 566

Protein: 59g

Carbs: 69g

Fat: 6g

Berry Beetsicle Smoothie

Preparation time: 3 minutes

Servings: 1

Ingredients:

- 1/2 cup peeled and diced beets
- 1/2 cup frozen raspberries
- 1 frozen banana
- 1 tablespoon maple syrup
- 1 cup unsweetened soy or almond milk

Directions:

Combine all theingredients in a blender and blend until smooth.

Nutrition:

Calories: 130,

Protein 9 g,

Fat 3 g,

Carbs 28 g,

Fiber 11 g

Green Breakfast Smoothie

Preparation time: 10 minutes

Servings: 2

Ingredients:

- 1/2 banana, sliced
- 2 cups spinach or other greens, such as kale
- 1 cup sliced berries of your choosing, fresh or frozen
- 1 orange, peeled and cut into segments
- 1 cup unsweetened non-dairy milk
- 1 cup ice

Directions:

In a blender, combine all the **Ingredients:**.

Starting with the blender on low speed, begin blending the smoothie, gradually increasing blender speed until smooth.

Serve immediately.

Nutrition:

Calories: 100, Protein 4 g, Fat 3 g, Carbs 20 g, Fiber 10 g

Blueberry Lemonade Smoothie

Preparation time: 5 minutes

Servings: 1

Ingredients:

- 1 cup roughly chopped kale
- 3/4 cup frozen blueberries
- 1 cup unsweetened soy or almond milk
- Juice of 1 lemon
- 1 tablespoon maple syrup

Directions:

Combine all theingredients in a blender and blend until smooth. Serve immediately.

Nutrition:

Calories: 95,

Protein 5 g,

Fat 6 g,

Carbs 22 g,

Fiber 11 g

Berry Protein Smoothie

Preparation time: 5 minutes

Servings: 1

Ingredients:

- 1 banana
- 1 cup fresh or frozen berries
- 3/4 cup water or nondairy milk, plus more as needed
- 1 scoop plant-based Protein powder
- 3 ounces silken tofu
- 1/4 cup rolled oats, or ½ cup cooked quinoa
- Additions
- 1 tablespoon ground flaxseed or chia seeds
- 1 handful fresh spinach or lettuce, or 1 chunk cucumber
- Coconut water to replace some of the liquid

Directions:

In a blender, combine the banana, berries, water, and your choice of Protein. Add any additioningredients as desired. Purée until smooth and creamy, about 50 seconds.

Add a bit more water if you like a thinner smoothie.

Nutrition:

Calories: 180,

Protein 18 g,

Fat 5 g,

Carbs 30 g,

Fiber 11 g

Chia Seed Smoothie

Preparation time: 5 minutes

Servings: 3

Ingredients:

- 1/4 teaspoon cinnamon
- 1 tablespoon ginger, fresh & grated
- Pinch cardamom
- 1 tablespoon chia seeds
- 2 medjool dates, Pitted
- 1 cup alfalfa sprouts
- 1 cup water
- 1 banana
- 1/2 cup coconut milk, unsweetened

Directions:

Blend everything together until smooth. Serve immediately.

Nutrition:

Calories: 210, Protein 8 g, Fat 9 g, Carbs 25g, Fiber 10 g

Mango with carrot Smoothie

Preparation time: 5 minutes

Servings: 3

Ingredients:

- 1 carrot, peeled & chopped
- 1 cup strawberries
- 1 cup water
- 1 cup peaches, chopped
- 1 banana, frozen & sliced
- 1 cup mango, chopped

Directions:

Blend everything together until smooth. Serve immediately.

Nutrition:

Calories: 240,

Protein 5 g,

Fat 3 g,

Carbs 70 g,

Fiber 13 g

The Super Green

Preparation time: 10 minutes

Cooking time: 0 minutes

Servings: 1

Ingredients:

- 1 tablespoon agave nectar
- 1 bunch kale, spinach, Swiss chard or combination
- 1 bunch cilantro
- 2 cucumbers, chopped and peeled
- 1 lime, peeled
- 1 lemon, outer yellow peeled
- 1 orange, peeled
- 1/2 cup ice

Directions:

Add all the listedingredients to a blender

Blend until you have a smooth and creamy texture

Serve chilled and enjoy!

Nutrition:

Calories: 3180

Fat: 15g

Carbohydrates: 8g

Protein: 5g

The Wrinkle Fighter

Preparation time: 10 minutes

Cooking time: 0 minutes

Servings: 1

Ingredients:

- 2 brazil nuts
- 1 tablespoon flaxseeds
- 1 orange, peeled and cut in half
- 2 cups wild blueberries, frozen
- 2 cups kale, roughly chopped
- 1 1/2 cups cold coconut water

Directions:

Add all the listedingredients to a blender

Blend until you have a smooth and creamy texture

Serve chilled and enjoy!

Nutrition:

Calories: 180; Fat: 15g; Carbohydrates: 8g; Protein: 5g

The Anti-Aging Turmeric and Coconut Delight

Preparation time: 10 minutes

Cooking time: 0 minutes

Servings: 1

Ingredients:

- 1 tablespoon coconut oil
- 2 teaspoons chia seeds
- 1 teaspoon ground turmeric
- 1 banana, frozen
- 1/2 cup pineapple, diced
- 1 cup of coconut milk

Directions:

Add all the listedingredients to a blender

Blend until you have a smooth and creamy texture

Serve chilled and enjoy!

Nutrition:

Calories: 430; Fat: 30g; Carbohydrates: 10g; Protein: 7g

The Anti-Aging Superfood Glass

Preparation time: 10 minutes

Cooking time: 0 minutes

Servings: 1

Ingredients:

- Water as needed
- 1/2 cup unsweetened nut milk
- 1-2 scoops vanilla Whey Protein
- 1 tablespoon unrefined coconut oil
- 1 tablespoon chia seeds
- 1 tablespoon almond butter
- 1/4 cup frozen blueberries
- 1/2 stick frozen acai puree

Directions:

Add all the listedingredients to a blender

Blend until you have a smooth and creamy texture

Serve chilled and enjoy!

Nutrition:

Calories: 162

Fat: 14g

Carbohydrates: 10g

Protein: 3g

The Glass of Glowing Skin

Preparation time: 10 minutes

Cooking time: 0 minutes

Servings: 1

Ingredients:

- 1/2 avocado, sliced
- 2 cups kale
- 1 cup mango, chopped
- 1 cup pineapple, chopped
- 2 frozen bananas, peeled and sliced
- 1/2 cup of coconut water
- 1 tablespoon flax

Directions:

Add all the listedingredients to a blender

Blend until you have a smooth and creamy texture

Serve chilled and enjoy!

Nutrition:

Calories: 430; Fat: 40g; Carbohydrates: 20g; Protein: 10g

The Feisty Goddess

Preparation time: 10 minutes

Cooking time: 0 minutes

Servings: 1

Ingredients:

- 1 cup unsweetened almond milk
- 2 tablespoons lemon juice
- 2 tablespoons avocado, peeled and pit removed
- 1 tablespoon sunflower seeds
- 1/2 medium banana, ripe
- 1 cup packed spinach

Directions:

Add all the listedingredients to a blender

Blend until you have a smooth and creamy texture

Serve chilled and enjoy!

Nutrition:

Calories: 401; Fat: 42g; Carbohydrates: 4g; Protein: 2g

Smoothies 3

The Breezy Blueberry

Preparation time: 10 minutes

Cooking time: 0 minutes

Servings: 1

Ingredients:

- Handful of mint
- 1 teaspoon chia seeds
- 1 tablespoon lemon juice
- 1 cup of coconut water
- 1 cup strawberries
- 1 cup blueberries

Directions:

Add all the listedingredients to a blender

Blend until you have a smooth and creamy texture

Serve chilled and enjoy!

Nutrition:

Calories: 169; Fat: 13g; Carbohydrates: 11g; Protein: 6g

Powerful Kale and Carrot Glass

Preparation time: 10 minutes

Cooking time: 0 minutes

Servings: 1

Ingredients:

- 1 cup of coconut water
- Lemon juice, 1 lemon
- 1 green apple, core removed and chopped
- 1 carrot, chopped
- 1 cup kale

Directions:

Add all the listedingredients to a blender

Blend until you have a smooth and creamy texture

Serve chilled and enjoy!

Nutrition:

Calories: 116; Fat: 5g; Carbohydrates: 14g; Protein: 6g

A Tropical Glass of Chia

Preparation time: 10 minutes

Cooking time: 0 minutes

Servings: 1

Ingredients:

- 1 cup coconut water
- 1 tablespoon chia seeds
- 1 cup pineapple, sliced
- 1/2 cup mango, sliced

Directions:

Add all the listedingredients to a blender

Blend until you have a smooth and creamy texture

Serve chilled and enjoy!

Nutrition:

Calories: 90

Fat: 5g

Carbohydrates: 11g

Protein: 4g

Simple Anti-Aging Cacao Dream

Preparation time: 10 minutes

Cooking time: 0 minutes

Servings: 1

Ingredients:

- 1 cup unsweetened almond milk
- 1 tablespoon cacao powder
- 6 strawberries
- 1 banana

Directions:

Add all the listedingredients to a blender

Blend until you have a smooth and creamy texture

Serve chilled and enjoy!

Nutrition:

Calories: 220

Fat: 9g

Carbohydrates: 20g

Protein: 6g

The Gut Heavy Smoothie

Preparation time: 10 minutes

Cooking time: 0 minutes

Servings: 1

Ingredients:

- 2-3 cups spinach leaves
- 1/2 cup frozen blueberries, unsweetened
- 1 serving aloe vera leaves
- 1/2 cup plain full-Fat yogurt
- 1 scoop Pinnaclife prebiotic Fiber
- 1 and 1/2 tablespoons coconut oil, unrefined
- 1 tablespoon chia seeds
- 1 tablespoon hemp hearts
- 1 cup of water

Directions:

Add listedingredients to a blender

Blend until you have a smooth and creamy texture

Serve chilled and enjoy!

Nutrition:

Calories: 409; Fat: 33g; Carbohydrates: 8g; Protein: 12g

Fresh Purple Fig Smoothie

Preparation time: 5 minutes

Cooking time: 0 minutes

Servings: 2

Ingredients:

- 1 fig
- 1 cup grapes
- 1/2 teaspoon maqui powder
- 1 cup of water
- 1 pear, chopped

Directions:

Add all the listedingredients to a blender

Blend until you have a smooth and creamy texture

Serve chilled and enjoy!

Nutrition:

Calories: 136; Fat: 4g; Carbohydrates: 28g; Protein: 3g

Mesmerizing Strawberry and Chocolate Shake

Preparation time: 10 minutes

Cooking time: 0 minutes

Servings: 1

Ingredients:

- 1/2 cup strawberry, sliced
- 1 tablespoons coconut flake, unsweetened
- 1 and 1/2 cups of water
- 1/2 cup heavy cream, liquid
- 1 tablespoon cocoa powder
- 1 pack stevia

Directions:

Add all the listedingredients to a blender

Blend on medium until you have a smooth

Serve chilled and enjoy!

Nutrition:

Calories: 470; Fat: 46g; Carbohydrates: 15g; Protein: 4g

The Strawberry Almond Smoothie

Preparation time: 10 minutes

Cooking time: 0 minutes

Servings: 1

Ingredients:

- 1/4 cup frozen strawberries, unsweetened
- 16 ounces unsweetened almond milk, vanilla
- 1 scoop vanilla whey Protein
- 1 pack stevia
- 4 ounces heavy cream

Directions:

Add all the listedingredients into your blender

Blend until smooth

Serve chilled and enjoy!

Nutrition:

Calories: 304; Fat: 25g; Carbohydrates: 7g; Protein: 15g

Hazelnut and Coconut Medley

Preparation time: 10 minutes

Cooking time: 0 minutes

Servings: 1

Ingredients:

- 1/4 cup hazelnuts, chopped
- 1/2 cup of coconut milk
- 1 pack stevia
- 1 and 1/2 cups of water

Directions:

Add all the listedingredients into your blender

Blend until smooth

Serve chilled and enjoy!

Nutrition:

Calories: 457; Fat: 46g; Carbohydrates: 12g; Protein: 7g

Overloaded Hazelnut and Mocha Shake

Preparation time: 10 minutes

Cooking time: 0 minutes

Servings: 1

Ingredients:

- 1-ounce Hazelnuts
- 2 cups brewed coffee, chilled
- 1 tablespoon MCT oil
- 2 tablespoons cocoa powder
- 1-2 packet Stevia, optional

Directions:

Add all the listedingredients into your blender

Blend until smooth

Serve chilled and enjoy!

Nutrition:

Calories: 325; Fat: 33g; Carbohydrates: 12g; Protein: 6.8g

Conclusion

Thank you for making it to the end. Smoothies are a great way to pack a lot of nutrients into one drink and to help people meet their daily nutritional requirements. You can make smoothies with any type of fruits and vegetables, and you can even add healthy and nutritious ingredients like chia seeds, flaxseeds, and hemp seeds.

Smoothies are delicious and can be a super convenient and quick meal. They're easy to make and come together quickly, and you can make a smoothie that you can enjoy for breakfast, lunch, or dinner.

Whether you are completely new to the world of Smoothies or just learning to explore new areas, the first thing that you should know about Smoothie making are the components that you need to have in every drink.

So, whether you are only making your Smoothie for a quick snack or breakfast, always try to incorporate the following components:

- Liquid

- Fat

- Protein

- Fiber

Fat, Protein and Fiber will help you to enhance the power of your Smoothie to keep you energized throughout the day, and it will help you to stay full and satisfied.

On the other hand, it will also provide you with all the valuable macronutrients that you may need.

Just in case you are wondering, fruits, nuts, vegetables, seeds are all amazing sources of fiber, protein, and fat.

Additional sources of protein include protein powders, beans and also certain vegetables.

You can also find good healthy fats in oils, such as coconut oil, flax, hemp, chia or even olive oil, as well as ghee, nut/seed kinds of milk.

And lastly, we come to liquid. This is the base of your Smoothie that will help you to blend your smoothie easily and aid in digestion, circulation, hydration, skin health and even nutrient absorption, all while flushing out your body and detoxing it.

Water is possibly the cheapest and most convenient option when it comes to the liquid base, but you can always opt for coconut water, seed/nut milk or even 100% fruit juice.

CPSIA information can be obtained
at www.ICGtesting.com
Printed in the USA
BVHW091932060721
611240BV00005B/487

9 781801 743853